Anti Cancer Diet Book

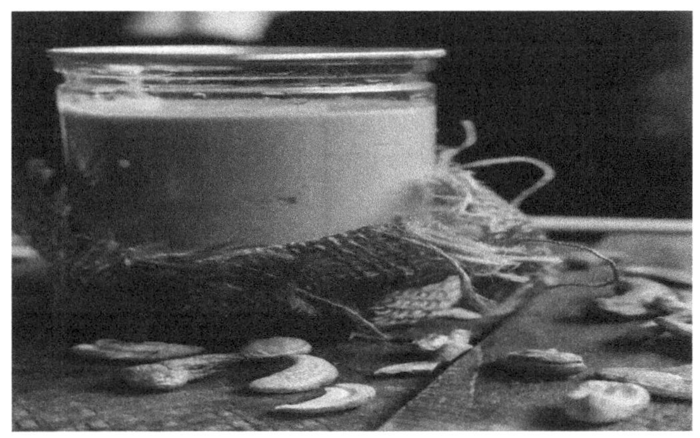

The Complete Anti Cancer Diet
(Whole Food) Cookbook for
Beginners

ISAAC HENDRICKS

Table of Contents

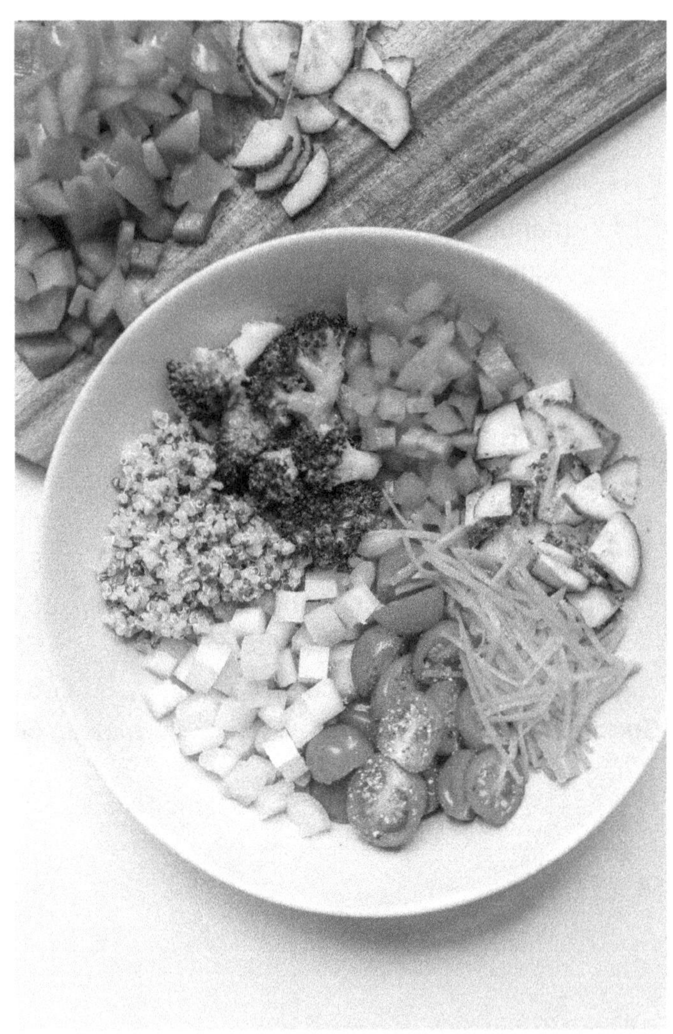

INTRODUCTION

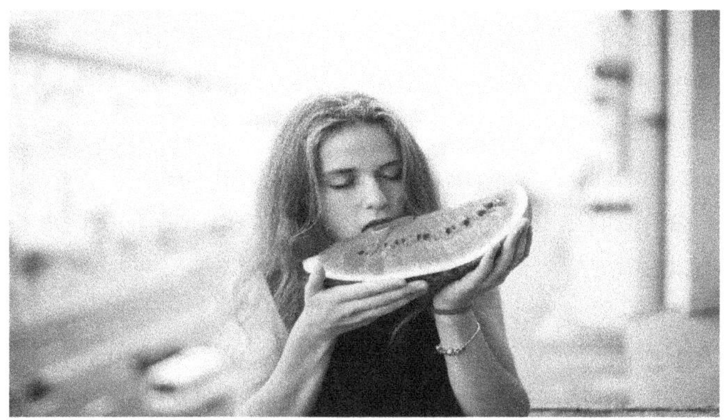

Recognising the Relationship between Nutrition and Cancer.

Cancer is a leading cause of death worldwide, with thousands of people diagnosed with the condition each year. While there are numerous factors that contribute to the development of cancer, research has shown that the relationship between nutrition and cancer is undeniable. Proper nutrition can significantly reduce the risk of cancer, while a poor diet can increase the likelihood of developing the disease.

The primary way in which nutrition affects the development of cancer is through obesity.

Obesity is a major risk factor for numerous types of cancer, including breast, colon, and pancreatic cancer. A diet that is high in calories, saturated fats, and sugars can lead to weight gain and increase the risk of developing cancer. In contrast, a diet that is rich in fruits, vegetables, and whole grains can help maintain a healthy weight and reduce the risk of cancer.

Another way in which nutrition affects cancer risk is through the consumption of certain foods and nutrients. Research has found that certain foods, such as red and processed meats, are associated with an increased risk of cancer. Conversely, other foods, such as tomatoes and cruciferous vegetables, contain phytochemicals that can reduce the risk of cancer. Nutrients such as vitamin D and antioxidants also play a crucial role in protecting against cancer.

Overall, research has consistently demonstrated the strong relationship between nutrition and cancer. A healthy diet that is rich in fruits, vegetables, and whole grains and low in processed and high-fat foods can significantly reduce the risk of developing cancer. It is important that individuals take a proactive approach to their diet and make informed choices to reduce their risk of cancer.

Why an Anti Cancer Diet is Important

An anti-cancer diet is important because it involves the consumption of foods that can potentially reduce the risk of developing cancer or assist in cancer treatment. Cancer is a complex disease that develops when abnormal cells start to grow, divide uncontrollably and form a mass or lump. Although there is no single cause of cancer, several studies have indicated that diet plays a significant role in its development, propagation and progression.

An anti-cancer diet primarily focuses on eating foods that possess anti-inflammatory, antioxidant and immune-boosting properties. Such foods include fruits, vegetables, whole grains, nuts, seeds, legumes and lean proteins. These foods are abundant in nutrients, such as vitamins, minerals, fibre and phytochemicals, which all have specific roles in the body's cancer defence mechanisms. By including these nutritious foods in your diet, you can help prevent cancer or slow its progression.

Fruits and vegetables, in particular, are powerful cancer-fighting foods that provide a plethora of antioxidants that scavenge free radicals, molecules that can damage cells, leading to cancer. Other anti-cancer foods like whole grains and legumes are also loaded with fiber, which helps to reduce oestrogen levels in the body, a hormone that contributes to the development of various cancers.

In addition to eating an anti-cancer diet, reducing the intake of processed foods, refined sugars, red and processed meats, and alcohol is also crucial. These foods are known to promote inflammation, increase oxidative stress, and harm the immune system, all of which increase the risk of cancer.

In conclusion, a diet rich in anti-cancer foods, combined with a reduction in processed and unhealthy foods, can help prevent cancer development and improve the overall health of an individual. Adopting an anti-cancer diet can be a significant step towards reducing the risk of cancer and improving cancer treatment outcomes.

CHAPTER ONE

The Basics of Anti-Cancer Diet

What is an anti-cancer diet?

An anti-cancer diet refers to a way of eating that aims to reduce the risk of developing cancer or to support the treatment of cancer. It involves consuming specific foods that are believed to have cancer-fighting properties, while avoiding or minimising certain others that may be associated with an increased risk of cancer. The main principles of an anti-cancer diet typically include:

1. Emphasising fruits and vegetables: A diet rich in a variety of colourful fruits and vegetables is often recommended due to their high content of antioxidants, vitamins, minerals, and fibre, which may help protect against certain types of cancer.

2. Including whole grains: Whole grains, such as whole wheat, oats, brown rice, and quinoa, are preferred over refined grains as they retain their natural nutrients, fibre, and antioxidants.

3. Consuming lean protein: Choosing lean sources of protein, such as fish, poultry, legumes, and plant-based protein sources like tofu and tempeh, is recommended. Reducing the consumption of processed meats and limiting the intake of red meat is also advised.

4. Incorporating healthy fats: Opting for sources of healthy fats, like avocados, nuts, seeds, and olive oil, is encouraged, while minimising the consumption of unhealthy fats like trans fats and Saturated fats, which are commonly found in processed and fried foods

5. Limiting added sugars: Reducing the intake of sugary foods and beverages can help maintain a healthy weight and decrease the risk of obesity, which is associated with an increased risk of cancer.

6. Avoiding or limiting alcohol: Minimising alcohol consumption or avoiding it altogether is typically recommended, as excessive alcohol consumption has been linked to an increased risk of certain cancers.

It's important to note that an anti-cancer diet should be part of an overall healthy lifestyle, which includes regular exercise, maintaining a healthy weight, getting enough sleep, and not smoking. It is advisable to consult with a healthcare professional or a registered dietitian for personalised advice and guidance on adopting an anti-cancer diet.

The Principles of Anti Cancer Diet

An anti-cancer diet is one that includes foods and nutrition that can help reduce the risk of cancer or support cancer treatment and recovery. The following are some principles of an anti-cancer diet:

1. Eat plenty of fruits and vegetables: Fruits and vegetables are rich in antioxidants and phytochemicals that may protect against cancer. Make an effort to consume at least 5 servings of fruits and vegetables per day.

2. Choose whole grains: Whole grains contain fibre, vitamins, and minerals - all of which can help lower cancer risk. Choose whole-grain bread, pasta, rice, and cereals.

3. Reduce red and processed meat: Red and processed meat have been linked to an increased risk of certain cancers. Try to limit consumption of beef, pork, or lamb and choose lean meats like chicken or fish and plant-based proteins like beans, lentils, or tofu.

4. Avoid sugary drinks and processed foods: Sugary drinks and processed foods are high in calories, sugars, and unhealthy fats that can contribute to weight gain, inflammation, and other factors that increase cancer risk.

5. Choose healthy fats: Fats are important for your health, but choose healthy fats like olive oil, avocado, nuts, and seeds. Avoid trans and saturated fats, which are present in processed and fried foods.

6. Limit alcohol consumption: Drinking alcohol regularly has been linked to an increased risk of some cancers. Limit alcohol intake to no more than 1 drink per day for women and 2 drinks per day for men.

7. Stay hydrated: Drinking enough water can help flush out toxins and waste products from the body, reducing cancer risk.

Overall, an anti-cancer diet emphasises a variety of whole foods, limits processed and sugary foods, and encourages a healthy balance of macronutrients and hydration.

Nutrients' Function in Cancer Prevention

Nutrients play a crucial role in cancer prevention as they help in boosting the immune system and protecting cells from DNA damage. Some of the key nutrients that have been found to be effective in cancer prevention include:

1. Antioxidants: These are compounds that neutralise free radicals and prevent oxidative stress, which can damage cells and DNA. Examples of antioxidants include vitamins C and E, selenium, and beta-carotene.

2. Fibre: Fibre helps to reduce inflammation in the body, lower cholesterol levels, and support healthy digestion. Diets that are high in fibre have been linked to a reduced risk of colon cancer.

3. Omega-3 fatty acids: These healthy fats help to reduce inflammation and protect against cellular damage. Foods rich in omega-3 fatty acids include salmon, tuna, walnuts, and flaxseed.

4. Phytonutrients: These are plant-based compounds that have antioxidant and anti-inflammatory properties. Examples of phytonutrients include resveratrol in red grapes, curcumin in turmeric, and sulforaphane in broccoli.

5. Vitamin D: This essential nutrient helps to regulate cell growth and division, and a deficiency in vitamin D has been linked to an increased risk of certain types of Breast, colon, and prostate cancer are examples of cancers.

Incorporating nutrient-rich foods into your diet can help to lower your risk of developing cancer. A balanced diet that includes a variety of fruits, vegetables, whole grains, lean proteins, and healthy fats can provide your body with the nutrients it needs to fight off cancer cells and maintain optimal health.

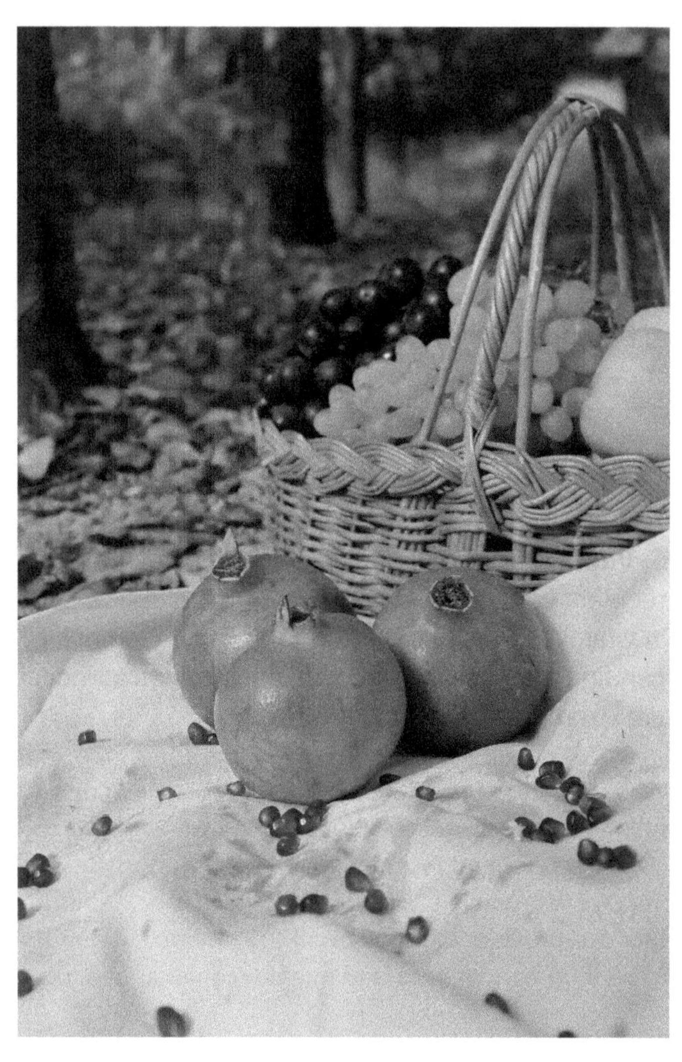

CHAPTER TWO

Foods to Avoid in an Anti-Cancer Diet

Foods that increase cancer risk

Cancer-causing foods are those that contain harmful compounds or chemicals that affect the DNA of our cells. These compounds or chemicals can be found in some foods that we commonly consume, such as processed meats, sugary drinks, foods with added sugars, and highly processed foods.

Processed meats such as bacon, sausages, hot dogs, and ham contain nitrates and nitrites, which are used as preservatives. These chemicals are known to increase the risk of colon cancer. Similarly, sugary drinks such as sodas and fruit juices contain high amounts of added sugars, which can lead to obesity and other health conditions that increase the risk of certain types of cancers.

Highly processed foods like frozen meals, snack foods, and fast food meals are often high in calories, unhealthy fats, and sodium. These types of foods can cause weight gain and increase inflammation in the body, which can increase the risk of several types of cancers.

Other foods that are known to increase cancer risk include red meat, alcohol, and charred or grilled foods. It is always recommended to focus on consuming a healthy diet rich in fruits, vegetables, whole grains, legumes, and lean proteins to reduce the risk of cancer and other chronic diseases.

The Dangers of Unhealthy Fats and Sugars

Unhealthy fats and sugars are known to contribute to a wide range of negative health effects in the long term. The dangers of unhealthy fats and sugars are numerous and pose a significant threat to individuals' health, particularly if consumed in large quantities.

The dangers of unhealthy fats include the risk of heart attacks, strokes, high blood pressure, and other cardiovascular diseases. This is because unhealthy fats contain high levels of cholesterol and can contribute to the formation of blockages in blood vessels, leading to restricted blood flow and ultimately, heart problems.

Saturated and trans fats, found in foods such as processed meats, fried foods, baked goods, and dairy products, are particularly harmful. These fats can raise LDL (low-density lipoprotein) cholesterol levels, which increase the risk of heart disease.

In addition to unhealthy fats, high levels of refined and added sugars can cause a host of adverse health effects. They contribute to obesity, type 2 diabetes, and other metabolic diseases by causing insulin resistance and inflammation in the body.

Consuming too much refined sugar, found in high-sugar drinks, candy, and baked goods, can lead to weight gain, tooth decay, and heart disease. Further, consuming large amounts of added sugars, found in processed foods such as ketchup and pasta sauces, can also lead to excess calorie consumption and negative impacts on health.

To combat the dangers of unhealthy fats and sugars, individuals should limit their intake of processed and fast foods and prioritise whole fruits, vegetables, whole grains, lean proteins, and healthy fats such as avocados and nuts. Adopting a balanced and varied diet can help individuals maintain a healthy weight, reduce the risk of heart disease and other chronic illnesses, and promote overall well-being.

Processed foods and their link to cancer

Processed foods, commonly found in supermarkets, are often high in sugar, salt, and fat. They are also often stripped of important nutrients as they undergo a manufacturing process. Studies have shown a concerning link between consumption of processed foods and cancer.

One of the most commonly used additives in processed foods is sugar. High levels of sugar consumption have been linked to an increased risk of cancer, particularly breast and colon cancer. This is thought to be due to the fact that sugar feeds cancer cells and promotes inflammation in the body, which can potentially lead to cancer.

Another common additive used in processed foods is sodium nitrate, which is used to preserve meats. This chemical has been linked to an increased risk of stomach cancer. Processed meats, such as deli meats and hot dogs, have been classified as a Group 1 carcinogen by the International Agency for Research on Cancer (IARC), placing them in the same category as tobacco and asbestos.

In addition to the additives used in processed foods, the manufacturing process itself can also contribute to cancer risk. Cooking foods at high temperatures, such as during the frying or grilling process, can lead to the formation of carcinogenic compounds.

To reduce the risk of cancer, it is recommended to limit the consumption of processed foods and choose whole, unprocessed foods whenever possible. Fruits and vegetables, whole grains, and lean protein sources are all examples. When buying processed foods, it is important to read the labels and choose options with fewer additives and preservatives.

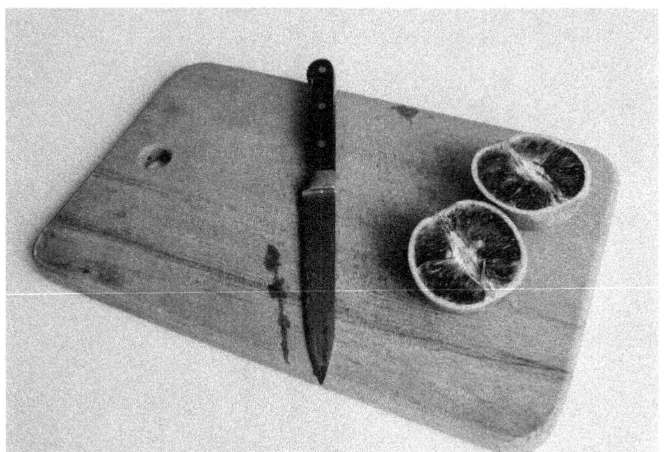

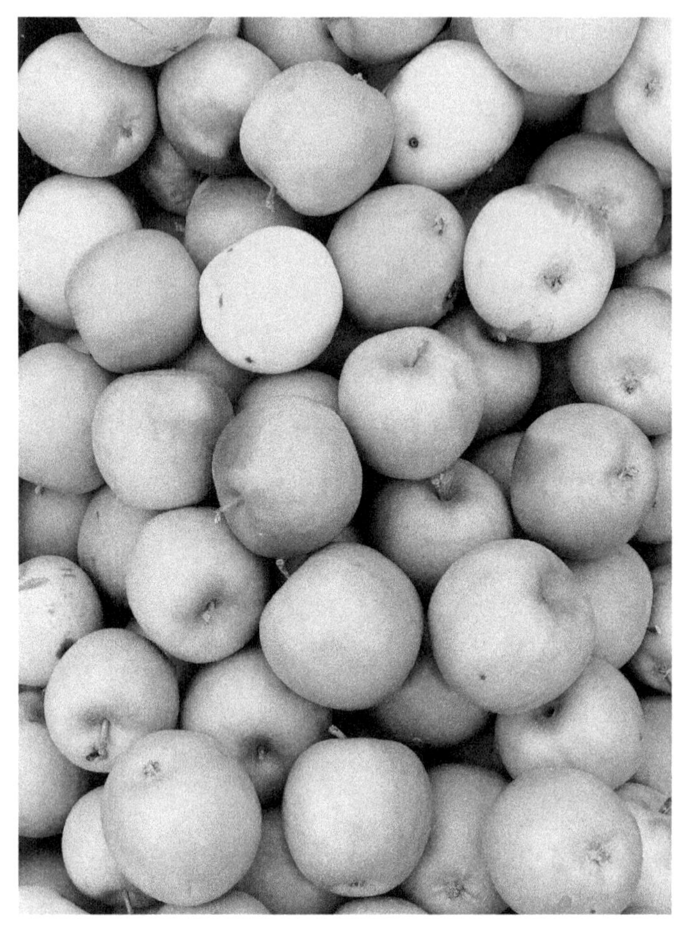

CHAPTER THREE

Foods to Include in an Anti-Cancer Diet

The importance of fruits and vegetables

Fruits and vegetables are essential to a healthy and balanced diet. They are high in vitamins, minerals, and fibre, which the body requires to function correctly. Here are some of the reasons why fruits and vegetables are important:

1. Nutrient dense:

Fruits and vegetables are rich sources of vitamins and minerals that are essential for good health. They are also low in calories, making them an excellent choice for weight management.

2. Improve digestion:

Fruits and vegetables are high in fibre, which helps to improve digestion, prevent constipation, and reduce the risk of colon cancer.

3. Boost immunity:

Fruits and vegetables are rich in antioxidants, which help to boost the immune system and prevent disease.

Eating a diet rich in fruits and vegetables has been associated with a reduced risk of chronic diseases such as type 2 diabetes, heart disease, and some types of cancer.

Fruits and vegetables contain antioxidants and vitamins that help to promote healthy skin and reduce the signs of ageing.

Overall, incorporating a variety of fruits and vegetables into your diet is essential for maintaining good health and preventing disease.

Whole grains, legumes, and nuts

Whole grains, legumes, and nuts are some of the most important food items in a healthy diet. They are packed with essential nutrients, fiber, and protein that are vital for maintaining good health and well-being.

Whole grains are unrefined grains that contain the whole grain kernel, including the bran, germ, and endosperm. They are rich in complex carbohydrates, fiber, vitamins, minerals, and antioxidants that can provide several health benefits, such as reducing the risk of heart disease, diabetes, and certain types of cancer. Examples of whole grains include brown rice, quinoa, barley, oatmeal, and whole wheat bread.

Legumes are the seeds or pods of plants in the pea family. They are an excellent source of plant-based protein, fiber, folate, potassium, and iron. Legumes can come in many different varieties, such as lentils, chickpeas, black beans, and kidney beans. They are a great addition to any dish and can be added to salads, soups, stews, and casseroles.

Nuts are small and nutrient-dense food items that are packed with healthy fats, protein, fiber, vitamins, and minerals. They are considered to be heart-healthy and can help with weight management. Examples of nuts include almonds, walnuts, pistachios, and cashews. Nuts can be a great snack or can be used as a topping for salads and oatmeal.

In conclusion, whole grains, legumes, and nuts are important components of a healthy diet. Including these food items in your meals can provide a range of health benefits and improve overall health and well-being.

The role of healthy fats and proteins in an anti-cancer diet

Healthy fats and proteins are essential components of an anti-cancer diet due to their numerous benefits. Some of these benefits include:

1. Reduced inflammation: Healthy fats such as omega-3 fatty acids and monounsaturated fats have anti-inflammatory properties that help to reduce inflammation in the body. Cancer development is connected to chronic inflammation.

2. Improved immune function: Proteins provide the building blocks for the immune system, and a diet rich in high-quality proteins such as fish, poultry, and legumes can help to improve immune function. A strong immune system is essential for fighting cancer cells.

3. Reduced insulin resistance: Insulin resistance is a risk factor for many types of cancer, and healthy fats such as those found in avocado and nuts can help to reduce insulin resistance.

4. Increased satiety: Foods high in healthy fats and proteins help to keep you feeling fuller for longer, which can help with weight management. Being overweight or obese puts you at risk for a variety of cancers.

Examples of healthy fats and proteins that are beneficial for an anti-cancer diet include:

- Fatty fish such as salmon, mackerel, and sardines
- Almonds, walnuts, and chia seeds are examples of nuts and seeds.
- Avocado
- Olive oil
- Legumes such as lentils and chickpeas
- Lean protein sources such as chicken and turkey
- Dairy items with low fat, such as yogurt and cottage cheese.

Overall, incorporating healthy fats and proteins into the diet can help to reduce the risk of cancer and improve overall health.

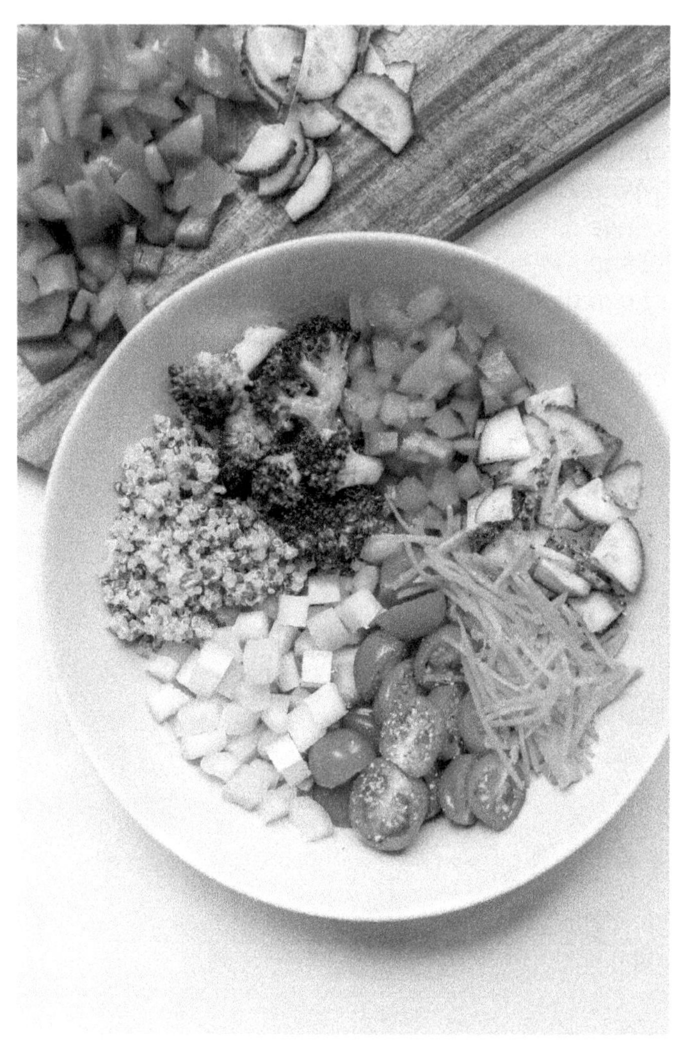

CHAPTER FOUR

Anti-Cancer Superfoods

Top anti-cancer foods and their benefits

1. Cruciferous Vegetables:

These include broccoli, cabbage, kale, and cauliflower, contain sulforaphane, a compound that reduces inflammation and oxidative stress, and helps protect against cancer.

2. Berries:

Blackberries, strawberries, blueberries, and raspberries contain powerful antioxidants like anthocyanins, which have been shown to protect against cancer.

3. Garlic:

Garlic contains sulfur compounds that have been shown to have anticancer effects, particularly against stomach and colorectal cancers.

4. Green Tea:

Green tea contains polyphenols, compounds that have antioxidant and anticancer properties. Studies have shown that drinking green tea can lower the risk of several types of cancers.

5. Turmeric:

Turmeric contains curcumin, a compound with potent anti-inflammatory and antioxidant properties. Curcumin has also been shown to have anticancer effects, particularly against breast, prostate, and colon cancers.

6. Dark Leafy Greens:

Dark leafy greens like spinach, kale, and Swiss chard are rich in antioxidants and anti-inflammatory compounds that can help protect against cancer.

7. Tomatoes:

Tomatoes are rich in lycopene, a powerful antioxidant that has been linked to a lower risk of prostate cancer.

8. Beans and Legumes:

Beans and legumes like lentils, chickpeas, and black beans are rich in fiber, protein, and nutrients that can help protect against cancer.

9. Nuts:

Nuts like almonds, walnuts, and pecans are rich in antioxidants, healthy fats, and other nutrients that can help protect against cancer.

10. Mushrooms:

Mushrooms contain compounds like beta-glucans, which have been shown to have anticancer properties. Some studies have also suggested that mushrooms may help boost the immune system and fight cancer.

Incorporating superfoods into your diet

Superfoods are nutrient-dense foods that offer vast health benefits to the body. Incorporating them into your diet can help improve your overall well-being, reduce the risk of chronic diseases, and boost energy levels. Here are some tips on how to easily incorporate superfoods into your diet:

1. Start by identifying the superfoods you like: Incorporating superfoods doesn't mean you should suddenly start eating foods you don't enjoy. Instead, choose the ones you like, and slowly incorporate them into your diet.

2. Experiment with new recipes: Look for recipes that use your favorite superfoods to create delicious and nutritious meals. For instance, if you love broccoli, you can search the internet for broccoli salad recipes to create a healthy meal.

3. Swap out unhealthy foods with superfoods: Replace processed foods, candy, and other unhealthy snacks with superfoods like nuts, berries, and avocados.

4. Add superfoods to your smoothies: Smoothies are an excellent way to get a combination of superfoods into your diet. Add berries, spinach, chia seeds, and other superfoods to your go-to smoothie recipe to make it even healthier.

5. Meal prep with superfoods: Meal prepping is an easy way to ensure you have healthy meals throughout the week. Try adding superfoods to your meal prep routine to provide your body with the nutrients and vitamins it needs.

In conclusion, incorporating superfoods into your diet may seem daunting at first, but it's a simple process once you begin. With these easy tips, you'll soon be on your way to a healthier, more energized you.

CHAPTER FIVE

Dietary Supplements for Cancer Prevention

The importance of vitamins in a cancer-fighting diet

The human body requires a wide range of vitamins and minerals to function properly, and many of these nutrients play a crucial role in supporting immune system function and fighting cancer. Vitamins such as vitamin C, D, E, and K have been shown to be particularly important in cancer prevention and treatment.

Vitamin C is a powerful antioxidant that can help protect cells from damage caused by free radicals, which can lead to cancerous cell growth. Vitamin D plays a critical role in immune system function and is believed to help prevent cancer by slowing or stopping the growth of cancer cells. Vitamin E is another important antioxidant that can help protect against cancer-causing agents, and vitamin K has been shown to help regulate cell growth and may reduce the risk of certain types of cancer.

While vitamins alone cannot prevent or cure cancer, a diet that is rich in these essential nutrients can help support overall health and bolster the immune system's ability to fight cancer cells. It's important to note that it's best to obtain vitamins through a healthy diet rather than through supplements, as certain vitamins can be harmful in excess. Consult with a healthcare professional to determine which vitamins you need and in what quantities.

Herbal supplements and their benefits

Here are some commonly used herbal supplements and their purported benefits:

1. Echinacea - boosts immune system and reduces symptoms of cold and flu
2. Milk Thistle - detoxifies the liver and protects it from damage
3. Ginkgo Biloba - improves memory and cognitive function
4. St. John's Wort - helps with symptoms of depression and anxiety
5. Turmeric - reduces inflammation and pain
6. Valerian root - helps with insomnia and anxiety
7. Saw Palmetto - improves prostate health
8. Garlic - lowers cholesterol levels and reduces the risk of heart disease
9. Ginger - reduces nausea and inflammation

10. Chamomile - promotes relaxation and reduces anxiety.

It's important to note that herbal supplements can interact with prescription medications and may not be suitable for everyone. Consulting with a healthcare professional is recommended before taking any herbal supplements.

Essential vitamins and minerals

Essential vitamins and minerals are important for maintaining overall health and preventing various diseases. Vitamins are organic substances that are necessary for the proper functioning of the body, while minerals are inorganic substances that the body needs for metabolic processes.

Here are some essential vitamins and minerals and their functions:

Vitamin A - Essential for maintaining healthy skin, vision, and immune system. It is found in foods such as liver, carrots, sweet potatoes, and broccoli.

Vitamin C - Helps in collagen production, wound healing, and iron absorption. It is found in citrus fruits, tomatoes, and leafy greens.

Vitamin D - Plays a vital role in bone health and immune function. It can be obtained through direct sunlight exposure and fortified foods such as milk and cereal.

Vitamin E- It is an antioxidant that safeguards cells against free radical damage. Nuts, seeds, and vegetable oils contain it.

Vitamin K- It is required for the clotting of blood as well as bone health. Leafy greens, broccoli, and soybeans contain it.

Calcium - Essential for bone and teeth strength, muscle contraction, and nerve function. It is found in dairy products, leafy greens, and fortified foods.

Iron - A crucial component of hemoglobin, which is responsible for carrying oxygen in the blood. It is found in red meat, spinach, and beans.

Magnesium - This mineral is essential for muscle and nerve function, as well as bone health. It can be found in nuts, seeds, and leafy green vegetables.

Potassium - Required for normal heart and muscle function. It is found in bananas, potatoes, and avocados.

Sodium - Aids in fluid equilibrium in the body, although excessive consumption can result in high blood pressure. It is found in processed foods and table salt.

In conclusion, consuming a balanced and varied diet is crucial for obtaining the essential vitamins and minerals needed for optimal health. However, if you are unable to get sufficient nutrients through diet alone, supplements may be necessary.

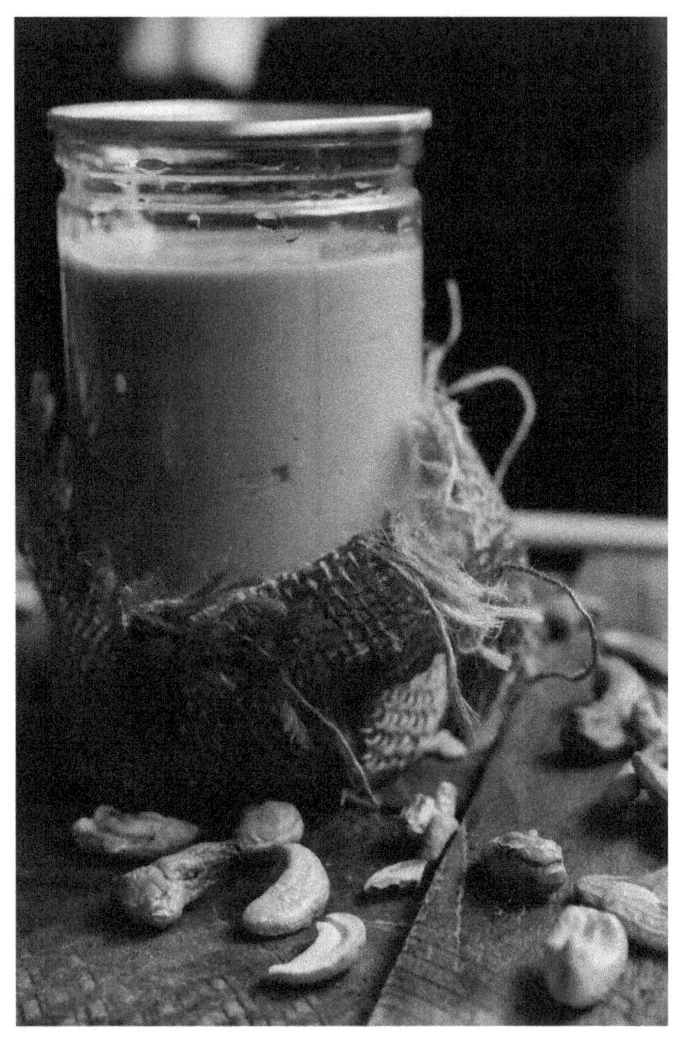

CHAPTER SIX

Lifestyle Changes to Support an Anti-Cancer Diet

Exercise and its role in cancer prevention and management

Regular exercise has a significant role in the prevention and management of cancer. A sedentary lifestyle is linked to a higher risk of developing cancer, and exercise can help prevent this by reducing body fat and improving metabolic function. Exercise is also known to improve the immune system, which can help reduce the risk of developing cancer as well as better manage cancer treatment.

A number of studies suggest that exercise can help prevent several types of cancer, including breast, colon, and prostate cancers. For example, a study published in the Journal of the National Cancer Institute found that women who engaged in moderate to vigorous physical activity had a lower risk of breast cancer than those who were inactive. Similarly, studies have suggested that exercising can reduce the risk of colorectal cancer by up to 25%.

Exercise also plays a vital role in managing cancer. People with cancer who exercise regularly have better quality of life, increased strength, and reduced fatigue, depression and anxiety. A study from the Journal of Clinical Oncology even showed that regular exercise in the weeks after surgery for breast cancer improved women's physical function and reduced the risk of lymphedema.

Exercise also helps to manage cancer in patients undergoing chemotherapy. Exercise has been found to reduce the toxic side effects of chemotherapy and improve patients' immune function. Exercise can help to reduce chemotherapy-related fatigue, one of the most common side effects, and help with nausea and other symptoms.

In conclusion, exercise plays a vital role in the prevention and management of cancer. Incorporating regular exercise into lifestyle and cancer treatment can help prevent cancer, improve patient quality of life, and better manage cancer symptoms. Exercise is an essential aspect of cancer treatment and should be encouraged for all cancer patients.

Stress management and relaxation techniques

Stress is a common part of everyday life, and can be caused by a variety of factors such as work, relationships or financial problems. If left unmanaged, stress can have negative effects on physical and mental health. It is therefore important to adopt stress management and relaxation techniques to help cope with stress and maintain a healthy body and mind.

There are various stress management techniques that individuals can practise to help reduce and manage stress. One technique is deep breathing exercises, which involves taking slow, deep breaths from your diaphragm. This can help to reduce muscle tension, lower blood pressure, and calm the mind. Meditation and mindfulness are other effective stress management techniques that involve focusing one's attention on the present moment. This can help to reduce racing thoughts, promote relaxation, and improve mental well-being.

Exercise is also a great way to reduce stress and manage anxiety. Regular physical activity releases endorphins, which are mood-boosting chemicals. Walking, yoga, and swimming are some forms of exercise that can promote relaxation and reduce stress. A healthy diet consisting of whole foods, fruits and vegetables, can also help reduce stress and anxiety. Avoiding caffeine, alcohol, and nicotine can help in reducing the stimulants that cause mental unrest.

In addition to stress management techniques, relaxation techniques can also help to reduce stress and promote relaxation. Some popular relaxation techniques include progressive muscle relaxation, guided imagery, and aromatherapy. Progressive muscle relaxation involves tensing and relaxing different muscle groups in the body, while guided imagery involves visualising a peaceful scene in your mind. Aromatherapy involves using essential oils such as lavender, peppermint, or chamomile to promote relaxation.

In sum, stress management and relaxation techniques are important tools in managing stress and promoting relaxation. Incorporating techniques such as meditation, exercise, deep breathing, and a healthy diet can help reduce stress and improve well-being. It is important to remember that each person's stress management and relaxation techniques may vary, and it is important to find techniques that work best for each individual.

The hazards of smoking and drinking alcohol

Smoking and drinking alcohol are two of the most dangerous habits that people can develop. These two habits can cause serious health problems and can lead to premature death. The hazards of smoking and drinking alcohol are numerous, and they affect nearly every system in the body.

Tobacco usage is a major cause of lung cancer, emphysema, and heart disease. The chemicals in cigarettes, such as tar and nicotine, can damage the lungs, heart, and blood vessels, leading to chronic lung disease, heart attacks, and strokes. Smoking also increases the risk of developing other types of cancers, including bladder, throat, and mouth cancers. In addition, smoking can cause infertility in men and women, as well as premature aging.

As for alcohol, it is a depressant that affects the brain's communication pathways, causing changes in mood, behaviour, and coordination. Drinking too much alcohol can lead to liver disease, high blood pressure, and even damage to the brain in extreme cases. Drinking alcohol in excess can also lead to addiction, accident and injury, and even death from alcohol poisoning.

Both smoking and drinking alcohol can also have negative effects on the social and emotional aspects of a person's life. Smoking can lead to isolation from non-smokers, and alcohol abuse can cause relationship problems, job loss, and financial hardship.

It is essential to understand the risks associated with smoking and drinking alcohol and take necessary measures to prevent harm to oneself. Avoiding these habits is the safest way to live a healthy and happy life. If one is already addicted to smoking or drinking, they should seek professional help to overcome their addiction and improve their overall health and well-being.

CHAPTER SEVEN

Recipes for an Anti-Cancer Diet

Delicious and easy-to-make anti-cancer recipes

Some delicious and easy-to-make anti-cancer recipes that are recommended by nutritionists and health experts.

1. Broccoli Salad with Chia Dressing
Ingredients:
- 1 head of broccoli, chopped
- 1 red onion, sliced thinly
- 2 tablespoons of chia seeds
- 3 tablespoons of apple cider vinegar
- 1 tablespoon of honey
- 1 tablespoon of Dijon mustard
- Salt and pepper to taste

Instructions:
1. In a large bowl, mix broccoli and onion.
2. In a small bowl, whisk together chia seeds, vinegar, honey, and mustard.
3. Pour dressing over the veggies and toss well.
4. Season with salt and pepper to taste.

2. Baked Salmon with Lemon and Herbs
Ingredients:

- 4 salmon fillets
- 2 tablespoons of olive oil
- 2 tablespoons of minced fresh herbs (such as parsley, thyme, and basil)
- Juice of 1 lemon
- Salt and pepper to taste

Instructions:
1. Preheat the oven to 375°F.
2. Place salmon in a baking dish and brush with olive oil.
3. Sprinkle herbs over the top, squeezing lemon juice over the salmon.
4. Season with salt and pepper.
5. Bake for 15-20 minutes, or until thoroughly done.

3. Berry Smoothie with Turmeric
Ingredients:
- 1 cup of mixed frozen berries
- 1 banana
- 1 tablespoon of turmeric powder
- 1 tablespoon of chia seeds
- 1 cup of unsweetened almond milk

Instructions:
1. In a high-speed blender, combine all of the ingredients until smooth.
2. Pour into a glass and enjoy!

These recipes are not only delicious but also packed with nutrients and anti-cancer properties that can help fight against cancer. By incorporating these meals into your daily diet, you can enjoy a healthy and vibrant lifestyle.

Smoothies, juices, salads, and entrees

Smoothies, juices, salads, and entrees are all popular food options that are known for their health benefits. These foods are not only delicious and nutritious, but they can also help you achieve your fitness and health goals.

Smoothies and juices are perfect for people who want to get a quick and refreshing source of nutrients. Smoothies are often made with fresh fruits and vegetables and can be combined with yoghourt or milk to create a creamy and filling drink. Juices are also made with fruits and vegetables and are perfect for those who want a quick boost of vitamins and antioxidants.

Salads are another healthy food option that can be enjoyed as a main meal or a side dish. Salads are made with fresh greens and can be topped with a variety of fruits, vegetables, nuts, and seeds. They are perfect for people who want a healthy and low-calorie meal option that is also packed with vitamins and minerals.

Entrees are the main course at any meal and can be made with a variety of healthy ingredients. Some popular entrees include grilled fish or chicken, roasted vegetables, and quinoa bowls.

These dishes are not only delicious, but they are also packed with protein, fibre, and healthy fats.

Overall, smoothies, juices, salads, and entrees are all excellent food options that can provide numerous health benefits. Whether you are trying to lose weight, maintain a healthy diet, or boost your energy levels, these foods are perfect for helping you achieve your goals.

Practical meal planning tips and sample menus

These are some practical tips on meal planning that can be done weekly to make mealtime easier and less stressful.

1. Plan your meals for the week ahead. Before the start of the week, plan which meals you will cook for breakfast, lunch, and dinner. Making a meal plan can help you save time, money, and effort. You can also make a grocery list to ensure that you have everything you need in your pantry, refrigerator, and freezer.

2. Choose easy meals for busy days.
On busy days, it's better to cook meals that are quick and easy to prepare. You can make use of your leftovers or cook one-pot meals such as soups, stews, or pasta dishes.

3. Use a slow cooker.

Slow cookers are great for busy days because you can prepare your meals in the morning and let them cook all day without constant supervision. You can come home to a hot and delicious meal that's ready to eat.

4. Prep your ingredients ahead of time.

Preparing your ingredients ahead of time can save you a lot of time and effort. You can wash, chop, and store your vegetables and meat a day or two ahead of time.

5. Cook in batches.

Cooking in batches will help you save time in the long run. You can cook more than you need and freeze the rest for later.

Sample Menu

Monday:

Breakfast: Greek yogurt with granola and fresh fruit

Lunch: Tuna salad sandwich on whole-grain bread with carrot sticks

Dinner: Grilled chicken breasts with garlic and rosemary, roasted potatoes, and green beans

Breakfast: Scrambled eggs, whole-wheat toast, and orange juice

Lunch: Leftover grilled chicken breasts with mixed greens and cherry tomatoes

Dinner: Baked fish fillet with lemon and herbs, brown rice, and steamed broccoli

Wednesday:

Breakfast: Oatmeal with banana and almonds

Lunch: Ham and swiss cheese sandwich on whole-grain bread with apple slices

Dinner: Beef stir-fry with bell peppers and broccoli over white rice

Thursday:

Breakfast: Greek yogurt with honey and chopped almonds

Lunch: Leftover beef stir-fry over quinoa with cucumber salad

Dinner: Spaghetti with marinara sauce, meatballs, and garlic bread

Breakfast: Scrambled eggs, black beans, cheese, and salsa in a breakfast burrito

Lunch: Veggie wrap with hummus, carrots, cucumber, and spinach

Dinner: Grilled salmon with lemon and herbs, roasted potatoes, and asparagus

Saturday:

Breakfast: Belgian waffles with fresh fruit and whipped cream

Lunch: Chicken Caesar salad with croutons

Dinner: Vegetable lasagna with garlic bread and mixed green salad

Sunday:

Breakfast: Breakfast casserole with bacon, eggs, cheese, and spinach

Lunch: Leftover vegetable lasagna with mixed green salad

Dinner: Roasted turkey breast with gravy, stuffing, mashed potatoes, and cranberry sauce.

Meal planning is a crucial aspect of leading a healthy lifestyle, especially for those who are fighting cancer. Planning ahead and making mindful food choices can help boost the immune system and promote overall well-being. Here are some practical tips and sample menus to consider:

1. Make a list of anti-cancer foods:

Anti-cancer foods include fruits, vegetables, whole grains, lean protein, and healthy fats. Incorporating these foods into your diet can help prevent cancer and reduce the risk of recurrence. Some examples include:

- Cruciferous vegetables (broccoli, cauliflower, kale)
- Berries (blueberries, raspberries)
- Leafy greens (spinach, arugula, kale)
- Whole grains (brown rice, quinoa)
- Lean protein (chicken, fish, legumes)
- Healthy fats (olive oil, avocado, nuts)

2. Plan meals in advance:

Meal planning ahead of time can help you eat a balanced and nutritious diet. Make a weekly meal plan and write out a grocery list to make shopping easier. Meal prepping can also be helpful, as it allows you to have healthy meals ready to eat throughout the week.

3. Use herbs and spices:

Herbs and spices not only add flavour to meals but also have anti-inflammatory and anti-cancer properties. Some examples include:

- Turmeric
- Garlic
- Ginger
- Cinnamon
- Oregano

Sample menus:

Breakfast:
- Greek yoghourt with berries and granola
- Oatmeal with banana slices and almond butter
- Avocado toast with scrambled eggs

Lunch:
- Salad with mixed greens, grilled chicken, tomatoes, and avocado
- Quinoa bowl with roasted vegetables and chickpeas
- Turkey and cheese wrap with a side of raw vegetables

Dinner:
- Baked salmon with roasted vegetables and brown rice
- Stir-fried chicken with broccoli and carrots
- Lentil soup with a side salad

Snacks:
- Apple slices with almond butter
- Carrots and hummus
- Nut and dried fruit trail mix

In conclusion, meal planning is an important aspect of living a healthy lifestyle, especially for those fighting cancer. By incorporating anti-cancer foods, planning meals in advance, and using herbs and spices, you can create delicious and nutritious meals that support your health and well-being.

Conclusion

Cancer is a major health concern that affects millions of people worldwide. While there is no surefire way to prevent cancer, evidence suggests that dietary choices can make a significant difference in reducing the risk of developing cancer.

However, a balanced and mindful approach to an anti-cancer diet is essential because many popular diets are often low in vital nutrients or heavily restrict certain food groups, leading to nutritional imbalances or deficiencies.

A balanced and mindful approach to an anti-cancer diet focuses on consuming a variety of nutrient-dense foods, including fruits, vegetables, whole grains, lean protein sources and healthy fats. These foods are rich in essential vitamins, minerals and antioxidants that help protect the body's cells from damage and reduce the risk of developing cancer.

It is also important to maintain a healthy weight, as being overweight or obese is a significant risk factor for several types of cancer, including breast, colorectal, and kidney cancer. A balanced anti-cancer diet includes portion control and limiting highly processed, high-calorie foods that contribute to weight gain.

Furthermore, mindful eating practices, such as being aware of hunger and fullness cues, and eating slowly, can help in maintaining a healthy weight and avoiding overeating. Mindful eating also promotes enjoyment of food and allows for a deeper appreciation of its flavours and textures, leading to better digestion and nutrient absorption.

Living a healthier lifestyle requires a dedicated effort to make positive changes. It's not always easy to break old habits or adopt new ones, but it's certainly worth the effort in the long run. If you're ready to move forward with a healthier lifestyle, here are a few tips to consider:

1. Set reasonable goals:
When making goals, be practical. Instead of aiming to run a marathon within a few months of starting your new lifestyle, aim for smaller goals like walking daily for 30 minutes or making healthier food choices.

2. Focus on nutrition:
A healthy diet is essential to a healthy lifestyle. Incorporate more fruits, vegetables, lean proteins, and whole grains into your meals while reducing your intake of processed foods, saturated fats, and added sugars.

3. Exercise regularly:
Exercise is important for maintaining a healthy weight, building muscle, and reducing the risk of

chronic illnesses. Most days of the week, aim for at least 30 minutes of moderate exercise, such as brisk walking.

4. Practice stress management:
Chronic stress can contribute to a number of health conditions, so it's important to learn how to manage stress. Deep breathing, meditation, and yoga can all be beneficial.

5. Get adequate sleep:
Getting enough sleep is critical for optimum health. Aim for 7-9 hours of sleep each night and establish a relaxing nighttime routine to promote better sleep.

In addition to these tips, it's important to make gradual changes over time and to find activities and foods that you enjoy. A healthier lifestyle doesn't have to be boring or restrictive – it can be fun and fulfilling if you approach it with a positive mindset. Remember, progress over perfection – focus on making small but consistent steps in the right direction and you'll be on your way to a healthier lifestyle.

In conclusion, a balanced and mindful approach to an anti-cancer diet can have significant health benefits. By focusing on nutrient-rich foods, maintaining a healthy weight and practising mindful eating, individuals can reduce their risk of developing cancer and improve their overall health and well-being.

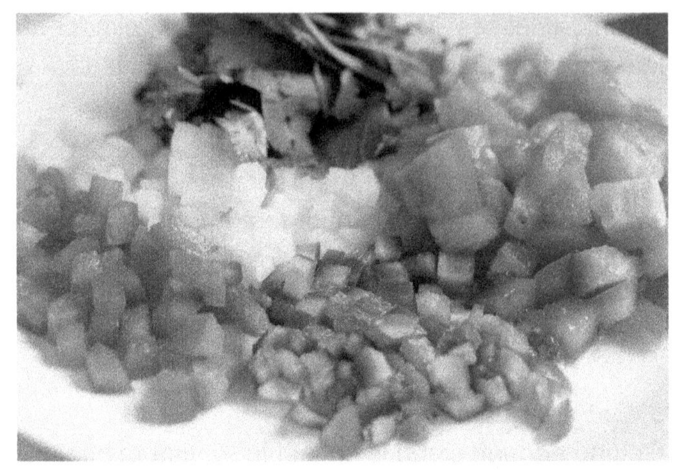